Does My Belly Look Big In This?

The Definitive Style Guide For Men

Sue Donnelly

First Published In Great Britain 2005
by www.BookShaker.com

© Copyright Sue Donnelly

Typeset in Trebuchet

For my husband Michael, with love.

CONTENTS

CONTENTS
FOREWORD
PREFACE

THE BOTTOM LINE 1

SUITS YOU, SIR 6
YOUR BODY SHAPE 9
GARMENTS TO SUIT YOUR BODY SHAPE 13
PROPORTIONS 17

THE ART OF ILLUSION... 19
SHORT LEGS/LONG BODY 19
SHORT BODY/LONG LEGS... 20
BEER BELLY 21
NARROW SHOULDERS 23
SMALL CHEST 23
SIZE IS EVERYTHING... 24
SHIRTS AND TIES... 29
COMBINING PATTERNS 32
ACT YOUR AGE... 32

LET'S FACE IT.. 35
OVAL 38
ROUND 38
HEART.. 39
PEAR 40
SQUARE.. 41
RECTANGLE.. 42
DIAMOND 43
TRIANGLE.. 44

H AIR TODAY GONE TOMORROW 45
T O BEARD OR NOT TO BEARD? 46
L OOKS GOOD ON YOU 46

COLOUR YOUR LIFE 48
D RESSING TO CHANGE YOUR APPROACH 53

SMART CASUAL - THE CONUNDRUM EXPLAINED 60

DRESSING FOR THE OCCASION 63
F ORMAL D INNERS 65
O THER B USINESS O CCASIONS 66
F UNERAL 67
J OB I NTERVIEW 67
C OURT A PPEARANCE 68
F IRST D ATE 68

WHAT YOUR BEST FRIEND WON'T TELL YOU 69
T HE E SSENTIALS 70
F ACING UP TO IT 74
S KIN T YPES 75
A CLOSE SHAVE? 76
S HAVING FOR PERFECT RESULTS 77
A FTER S HAVE 78
N OSE AND EARS 78
B ODY H AIR 80
H AIR P RODUCTS 81
H ANDS AND F EET 82
S MILE PLEASE 82
Y OUR BODY IS YOUR TEMPLE 83

WHO ARE YOU? 84
DRESSING A UTHENTICALLY 84

THE BARE ESSENTIALS 87

Pleased to meet you..87
"Daah-ling…"..89
Round the World in 80 days 90
Grooming 90
Body Language 92
Influencing Triangle 93
What A Poser! 94
Facial Expressions...94
What did you say? 95
Small Talk 96

PARETO IN YOUR WARDROBE 100
Shoes 105
Manage your wardrobe 105

LOOKING AFTER YOUR WARDROBE 108

NOW IT'S UP TO YOU 110

FOREWORD

I have interviewed many high profile successful people for our Internet TV Channel, www.expertsonline.tv and without exception they all acknowledge the critical importance that image has had at various moments on their journey to success.

From top broadcaster Eamonn Holmes to publicist Max Clifford and Health and Beauty guru Rosemary Conley, they all recognise the importance of dressing correctly to increase the chances of success.

Even though we are aware of this, generally speaking, men are pretty useless when it comes to choosing the clothes that suit them best. If I had a pound for every time my wife has said to me 'You are not going out dressed like that, are you?' I would be a billionaire by now. I do not believe I am stupid or moronic, but when it comes to matching up clothes, there appears to be a genetic flaw in males, which gets worse as we get older. It is one of life's mysteries, but nevertheless true.

This excellent style guide for men to read (and ladies should force them to read it) provides all the answers, with a title that should win awards before you even open it. The book provides us males with a long awaited insight into what to do and what not to do when it comes to dressing appropriately for the occasion – plus much more. There are no more excuses. This book is the solution. This is not a book to buy and then leave on a shelf gathering dust. It is a book that should be read and then re-read at least once every 3 months forever!

Wives and girlfriends the world over can now stop their years of frustration. Buy the book and, if all else fails, read it to your partner every night until he gets the message.

In my view, every ambitious male on the planet should have a copy of this book if they are serious about achieving their full potential. I recommend it to every man AND woman as a must have book.

Philip Crowshaw
FOUNDER AND CEO, EXPERTSONLINE.TV

PREFACE

When I first met Sue and realized she was an image consultant, my first thoughts were "why would I need one of those, after all I know exactly how to dress for work." As a business consultant it's straight forward -- there is only one approach. I wear a sharp suit, crisp shirt, bright tie and clean shoes, or had I got that wrong?

When Sue and I spoke, I started to realize that perhaps I was not as clever I as had first thought. Was my sharp, tailored image putting clients off and making them think that I was unapproachable, aloof, or just too 'corporate'? I started to think my style was perhaps not always appropriate for every environment in which I worked. I needed to become more flexible.

So I took stock, and tried to see myself as others might. What would I think if a pristinely dressed 6 feet 3 inch man was suddenly confronting me?

This experience prompted other thoughts which led me to speak to Sue again about casual wear. How many of us have been invited to a function where the dress code is described as 'Smart Casual'? I have never understood what that means and have always been scared of arriving either over or under dressed and looking the proverbial fool. The questions for me have been: should I wear a tie or is it open necked shirt; are jeans acceptable or should I wear formal trousers; must I wear a jacket and so on and so on.

Sue, being the professional she is, took all my concerns on board and applied a few simple guidelines. Not only has this made my life easier but the dilemma of dressing for business or social occasions has been addressed in this book in such a straight forward way that my concerns have disappeared. I can now relax and enjoy the function.

Thank you Sue, for writing such a compact yet enlightening book. 'Does My Belly Look Big In This?' is easily understood and gives men a set of ground rules to follow. There have been many style publications written for women over the years and, believe it or not, men are just as interested in getting it right – for ourselves and for our partners. This book enables you to do just that.

Colin Mogford
FOUNDER, ASHFORD MANAGEMENT LIMITED
colin@ashford-management.co.uk

THE BOTTOM LINE

"Style is the man himself"
Georges Louis Leclerc Buffon

Grooming and style. "Why bother?" you may ask. Aren't these the province of the female sex? You've done alright so far so why should you start to worry about it now?

Like it or not, you have an image whether you actively cultivate one or whether you don't. The way you present yourself to the rest of the world is the way you will be viewed. Whether that view is valid or not is up to you.

It has been said that if the first impression you make is the wrong one, it can take up to 21 subsequent meetings before the negative opinion of you is changed. So getting that first impression wrong can be expensive and time-consuming to rectify, whether it's a new client, a new boss or a new lady you're trying to impress.

We humans make snap judgements about people all the time. We are programmed to believe first what we see rather than what we hear, so our reference in this process centres round the visual clues we pick up.

Professor Albert Mehrabian highlighted in his book, *Silent Messages*, that what we actually say only accounts for very little (just 7%) of what people think of us. Non-verbal signals such as body language, eye contact, confidence, height, weight, colouring, clothing, hairstyles and accessories account for the remaining 93% and 55% of that concentrates on our visual appearance. So be careful before you dismiss your image out of hand.

Your casual, laid back look could be misconstrued as lazy and un-hygienic and could actually be getting in the way of job prospects and romantic success.

On the career front, Robert Half's research on promotional prospects also highlights the importance of having the correct image. Only 10% of potential success is concerned with actually *doing* the job well. It's assumed that anyone looking for promotion will already be skilled in their work. Image accounts for a substantial 30% with networking and personal promotion accounting for a massive 60%. Without the correct image, it is believed that you would struggle to promote yourself personally. So image is definitely not something that the career-minded man can afford to scoff at.

Women talk openly about clothes and makeup – it's part of their social upbringing – but it's often more difficult for the male population. Unfortunately, men, especially those over 40, don't have the luxury of being able to ask their mates, "does this make my belly look big?" so ultimately, you may not know what looks good. And just because a particular look, haircut or item of clothing suited you years ago, does not mean that your image is still appropriate today.

Women have always been aware that small changes can really affect how they feel and how they are perceived by others. A new hairstyle, a pair of glasses, a great handbag can all provide that feel good factor. In the corporate world, this is known as The Spiral of Success. When you look good, you feel good and your self esteem increases. In turn, this will enable you to project yourself with more conviction and confidence.

When you look your best others are drawn to you, so you are likely to gain more positive responses from work associates, family, friends and even strangers. From a business stance you are more likely to gain trust and respect with a resulting positive impact on your relationships and, ultimately, your bottom line.

So, as 90% of our bodies are covered by clothes for a good deal of the time, it would seem logical to dress ourselves in the best way possible. This book will help you to do just that. It will give you the chance to look at the basics in an unthreatening way. It will tell you things your best friend might not. It will help you to understand what really suits you, what to wear and when to wear it.

And, if you know you look good effortlessly, you'll feel good too, leaving you more time and energy to focus on the stuff that really matters to you.

So why is your image important? Because whatever you hope to achieve – new job, business success, great relationships, confidence, higher income or something else – all will become easier if you look the part. Trust me.

This book is for you if you want to:

1) Stay looking attractive, youthful and powerful in the working environment

2) Have more success with prospective love interests

3) Know how to look your best without losing touch with the real you

4) Age gracefully

5) Gain more authority, trust and respect

6) Make an impact at a special event - conference, job interview, court appearance

7) Know how to dress appropriately for any given occasion

8) Spend less time and money shopping because you just know what suits you

9) Make your wardrobe work for you

10) Actually enjoy the process of shopping

Finally, my promise to you is, that by the time you've finished this book, you'll be able to use your image as yet another tool for achieving the important things in your life!

SUITS YOU, SIR

*"Know first who you are and
adorn yourself accordingly"*
Epicetus, Greek Philosopher

Many years ago, the way a man dressed helped to identify where he belonged, in other words his tribe or family. Later, this evolved into the type of work he did and, in fact, still does to this day.

The military, police, clergy and legal profession for instance, all have a uniform which is instantly recognisable. Within these professions also exists a hierarchy, and the uniforms are designed so that each member is aware of rank and authority. Even football fans wear a 'uniform' enabling each person to easily identify their own team's supporters. It's like a password. If you are wearing the same clothes as me, then we have something in common – we are alike and I belong here.

Many politicians will change their normal attire to 'fit in' with a different audience. Eastern leaders may adopt a western dress, Prime Ministers and Presidents may sport a casual look, pop stars may wear a tuxedo. Wearing the right clothing creates a link with the people around you.

Pin striped suits were the province of the banking profession. The stripes in the fabric originally represented ledger lines used in book keeping. Today, the pin striped suit is still visible in the city, but has become more mainstream, certainly within the UK.

So, on the whole, the male race likes to fit in with its peers.

But, if you are a non-conformist who yearns to be different, beware, because there may be a price tag attached. Unless you are a style-icon such as David Beckham, or flamboyance personified, such as Sir Jonathan Ross or Sir Elton John, you may find yourself the subject of ridicule rather than a man of impeccable taste.

Now I didn't say you shouldn't remain an individual. I'll show you how you can express yourself with discreet little touches rather than an all out attack on other people's taste.

Not so long ago, men wore a suit to the office, confident they were wearing the right clothes for the job. These days, however, with the onset of a more casual working culture and 'dress down Fridays' looking the part has become much more of a challenge.

Many men no longer know what to do. It has become a bit of a quagmire when selecting clothing that is both appropriate and flattering. The tried and tested formula has gone.

Fundamentally it boils down to body shape. If you understand your shape, you are able to dress to best suit it, whatever the occasion. As many women have found to their cost, it is pointless buying an outfit because it looked good in a magazine, on someone else or on the rail. You need to know what suits YOU.

Exercise:

For this exercise, you will need a full length mirror. For optimum results, it's best to strip down to your underwear. Please also remember, that no one shape is better than another. All can be dressed to magnificence as long as the relevant style principles are applied. Just be honest with yourself.

YOUR BODY SHAPE

In essence, there are 3 main types of body shape:

Triangular – shoulders wider than hips

Rectangular – shoulders, waist and hips roughly equal

Contoured – a softer, more rounded look around shoulders, hips or stomach

Triangular

This body has wider shoulders than hips, so looks like an inverted triangle. You can be born with this type of body, or you may have defined your arm and shoulder muscles by working out at the gym or by regular physical work in your job.

Rectangular

Most men fit into this category. Weight doesn't matter as long as it doesn't reside around the stomach area, in which case move onto contoured. This shape is pretty well straight from top to bottom. This shape also gives the most choice when selecting clothes to suit it.

Contoured

Still fairly rectangular, this shape can be the result of putting on a few pounds, or being naturally well built. There is a softer edge to this shape but it doesn't always mean you are overweight. If you have sloping shoulders or wide hips, you will fit into this category. Likewise if you have a thick neck and/or your arms and legs are solid. If you have any kind of belly, this is where you belong.

All of the 3 shapes can be tall or short.

On the whole, a rule of thumb applies. If you are lean and angular, then stiff, starchy fabrics will best suit your body shape. If you are more contoured, then select fabrics with some 'give'. If you're not sure what I mean, imagine trying to wrap a golf ball in stiff paper! Rectangular shapes have the best of both worlds as either choice will look great.

The details and cut of your garments are also important. A contoured body will look better with a rounded hemline and softer lapels. An angular body, such as triangular, can go for sharp lapels and a straight hemline.

Vents at the back of your suit jacket are not really necessary today, unless you have a large backside.

Originally, these were provided so that the material could be spread along the back of a horse when the wearer was riding. If you do choose this type of jacket, the flaps of the jacket should still sit flat across the backside and not protrude.

Of course, a bespoke suit (one which is uniquely designed and tailored to your measurements) or a made-to measure one (a suit that is tailored to your measurements from an existing pattern) will always look great as it's made especially for you. There are cheaper, off the peg alternatives and as long as the fit and style suits your body, there is no reason why you shouldn't still look wonderful.

There are a number of different styles of suit. I am speaking broadly here, because all can have variations.

British. This is classic tailoring and may have the traditional vents. It's close fitting, single breasted and well structured with square shoulders. It may have two or three outside pockets, which may be flapped or angled, plus a pocket on the breast. It's also likely to have button hole and a four button cuff.

European. More modern and less structured than the British version. A roomier suit allowing ease of movement, without vents. It can be purchased as a double or single breasted suit. Slit or flapped pockets, a breast pocket, three or four button cuff and notched lapels. Shoulders may be slightly padded.

Modern. A look best left to younger men, footballers or those who work in the creative professions. Lots of buttons, no cuff buttons, exaggerated lapels and collar (could be a mandarin, stand up collar) are signs to look for.

All can be worn with waistcoats if required. Shirt sleeves should protrude between 1 and 4 centimetres below the cuff, depending on your scale, which we'll cover later. Cuff links should only be worn with a double cuffed shirt.

Below is a chart which reflects the best type of garments for each of the 3 shapes.

GARMENTS TO SUIT YOUR BODY SHAPE

	Triangular	Rectangular	Contoured
Suit/Formal Jackets	Little shoulder padding Single breasted Double breasted (if slim/long legged/tall) Wide or sharp lapels European style suiting Straight hemline Straight pockets	Some padding if added shoulder width required Single breasted. Double breasted (if slim/long legged/tall) Notched/peaked lapels European or British style (if under 5ft 8")	Adequate shoulder padding No vents (unless you have a large bottom) Single breasted Moderate lapels Contemporary style which is looser Rounded pocket flaps
Suit/Formal Trousers	Flat fronted Slim fit Wider legs	Regular fit Most styles suit	Pleated Relaxed fit

	if tall Turns up if jacket is double breasted	Single or double pleating (heavier figures)	
Casual Jackets	Blazer Bomber jacket with waist (probably looks best if under 40) Trench coat - belted Denim jacket (if under 40) Avoid boxy styles as added width at waist will fatten	Blazer Zip-front jacket Reefer Jacket Denim Jacket (probably looks best if under 40) Crombie	Pea jacket Sheepskin Coat or raincoat without structured tailoring Linen mix jacket Avoid anything double breasted
Casual Trousers	Stiff, straight	Most styles suit this	Cords

Trousers	legged jeans Flat fronted Wider legs if tall	shape	Softer weave jeans with baggy legs Chinos
Shirts	Tightly woven fabrics Avoid drapier fabrics Avoid long button down collars	Choice of drapey or starchy fabrics	Softer fabrics Avoid stiff fabrics and structured tailoring Avoid large/cutaway collars
Ties	Geometric designs e.g. stripes, checks as well as solid colour	Contoured or geometric pattern or solids	Paisleys, dots or solids
Tops	Fitted Shorter length	Straight shapes Moderate	Worn outside if tum is evident

	length	length	Longer length
	V-neck T-shirts	Round or V-neck T-Shirts	Drapey material Linen Avoid round neck T-shirts tucked in
Shorts	Trunks or shorts style trunks Knee length shorts - not too baggy	Shorts-style trunks Chino shorts Draw string shorts	Longer length trunks Drawstring shorts

You'll notice that I've mentioned blazers, but I'm not a big fan as I think they can look very dated. Triangular and Rectangular bodies can wear if tall, but team your blazer with chinos not grey flannels. Any double breasted jacket should always be fastened, as an open one looks untidy and can add bulk to your frame.

Talking of fastening, if you do wear a double breasted jacket it is customary to leave the bottom button undone. On a single-breasted jacket with 3 buttons you should leave the bottom button undone. You can also leave the top one undone, but never all three.

PROPORTIONS

Unfortunately, most men, whatever their age, do not have their ideal physique, with or without clothes. However, all is not lost. This next section is about cheating, and is the only part of the book dedicated to making you into something you're not!

It's all about lines. Those of you with an interest in art, architecture or maybe geometry will know there are 3 types:

1. Vertical – runs up and down

2. Horizontal – runs side to side

3. Diagonal – from top to bottom, left to right or vice versa

Our natural shape can be altered by using these lines so a different image is perceived by the viewer.

Vertical lines create length.

Horizontal and diverging lines create width.

Diagonal lines can shorten or lengthen. The more vertical the angle, the more length is created, the more horizontal, the more shortening the line.

Clever use of lines can make short legs appear longer, shoulders look wider, beer bellies look smaller and so on.

Fabric also plays a part, as does colour. Matt fabrics absorb light so make the body look slimmer. Shiny fabrics, on the other hand, reflect light and make the body look bigger. Dark colours also absorb light so a dark, matt fabric is a good choice to wear on a part of your body that needs to look thinner. Bright colours, such as red, have longer wave lengths so we see them first. It's no accident that red is used in traffic and car brake lights. So a shiny, bright red fabric is not always a good choice for hiding those little flaws.

Unfortunately, many football shirts have these two characteristics and definitely do not flatter any kind of beer belly.

The other major faux pas is the wallet, cigarettes, car keys etc kept in a back pocket of the trousers. This does nothing for your body shape it just adds bulk.

THE ART OF ILLUSION

*"Never trust a man with short legs -
brains too near their bottoms"*
Noel Coward, Playwright

The following are the main figure challenges that most of my male clients want to rectify. Using lines and fabric wisely, you can easily disguise the parts of your body that aren't so perfect.

SHORT LEGS/LONG BODY

Need vertical lines to create length.

This is not about the actual length of your leg but the proportionate size of your legs to the rest of your body.

Avoid turn ups on trousers as the horizontal line will shorten the leg. This also applies to tapered trousers. Make sure they are long enough. The front hem should break on the shoe and actually be a little longer at the heel.

Vertical stripes or a centre crease in your trousers give the illusion of length.

Try flip flops instead of sandals in the summer and definitely no socks.

A slight heel will make legs look longer.

Jackets should be no longer than bum length. Shorter jackets look good as long as you have no challenges round the hip or tum area.

This also applies to tops. Keep them shortish as long ones will shorten the legs even further.

Belts should match bottoms rather than tops.

Match your shoe colour to your trousers as this will elongate the leg.

Wear darker trousers and lighter tops, rather than the other way round.

SHORT BODY/LONG LEGS

Need horizontal lines to shorten the legs.

Turn ups on trousers are good as the horizontal line will shorten the leg. This also applies to tapered trousers. Make sure they are long enough. The front hem should break on the shoe and actually be a little longer at the heel.

Patterned trousers will shorten.

Sandals with horizontal fastenings will shorten the leg, as will shoes in a contrasting colour.

Jackets should be bum length and no shorter. Shorter jackets will make the legs appear even longer and the torso even shorter.

This also applies to tops. Keep them longer.

Belts, when going for a casual look only, should match tops rather than bottoms.

Wear lighter trousers and darker tops, rather than the other way round, unless you're under 5 feet 7 inches tall.

BEER BELLY

Needs vertical lines to create length.

A magazine editor once told me that if a men's magazine highlighted a feature on "How To Get A Six Pack" on the front cover, the circulation figures were sure to increase.

I'm guessing that for some of you, this is no longer an option. You like your couch potato life-style and the idea of the gym is a complete anathema.

My husband fits into this category – cuddly and proud of his belly, after all it cost a lot of money! The V-neck sweater is now one of his staple garments as it takes pounds of him. So give it a go and see the results for yourself.

Avoid any horizontal lines on your top half as they will widen and make you look fatter. Vertical lines will slim. This includes a ribbed knit.

Single breasted jackets and cardigans flatter but avoid double breasted jackets that will give the illusion of width.

Try braces, with your suit, for a funky look. Never wear braces and a belt together and never wear braces on casual trousers.

Wear shirts and tops worn out rather than tucked in.

Simple unstructured clothing rather than fitted will look better on you.

A waistcoat or sleeveless V-neck sweater in a dark colour will really reduce the size of your belly.

Make sure your tie is wide enough. A narrow tie will give the illusion of a larger body.

NARROW SHOULDERS

Need horizontal or diverging lines (V) to create width.

Wide lapels and shirt collars give the illusion of width.

Trench Coats with detail on the shoulder.

Shoulder pads in your suit tailoring.

Avoid excessive pleating around the waist as this will make your shoulders look out of proportion.

Go for bulkier sweaters.

Horizontal lines will make the chest area look larger.

Avoid raglan sleeves as this will make the shoulders look droopy and narrower.

Round necks look better than V-necks.

SMALL CHEST

Need horizontal lines to create width.

Horizontal lines will make the chest area look larger. .

Wear lots of thin layers rather than a thick bulky one.

Double breasted jackets add width, but avoid if you are short.

SIZE IS EVERYTHING

They say size doesn't matter but, in fact, where style is concerned, it does. The patterns you wear, the weight of the fabric, your accessories and even your tie width will look considerably better if the size reflects that of your body. If not, you're in danger of looking eccentric, over-powering or lost.

Look at the diagram below:

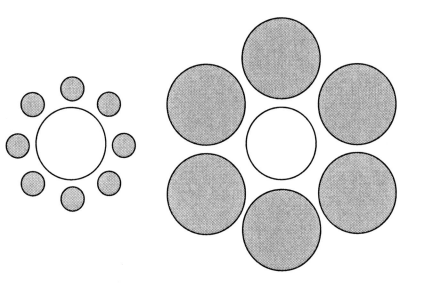

Which of the inner circles looks the smaller?

Actually the circles are the same size. The one surrounded by the larger circles only appears to be smaller because it is overshadowed by the larger ones.

If you wear clothes or patterns that are too large for you, you will appear swamped. Unfortunately, you will not look smaller just strange, so if you're larger than you'd like to be, then wearing patterns that are too big for your scale is not an easy alternative to proper eating and exercise! Conversely, if you wear too small a scale, you will look much bigger. While this may be OK for some guys, I can't imagine all of you would be happy about that.

Exercise:

Refer to the chart below to find your scale...

	LIGHT	AVERAGE	HEAVY
> 5 ft 11"	MEDIUM	LARGE	LARGE
5 ft 7" - 5 ft 11"	LIGHT	MEDIUM	LARGE
< 5 ft 7"	SMALL	SMALL	MEDIUM

Small scale

Fabric weights should be light. Suiting weight about 10oz.

Patterns should be small and also reflect your bodyline, for instance a small diamond-patterned tie would look great on a small scale, angular man.

Accessories, apart from specs which are covered later, should reflect both your scale and your bodyline. This means carrying a small briefcase and not a huge one. The latter will only make you look smaller.

Ties should be narrow.

Medium scale

Fabric should be of medium weight. Suiting about 12-14oz.

Patterns should be medium size and reflect your bodyline, for instance a medium paisley print tie would look great on you if you have a contoured body. Choose medium size checks or stripes if you're angular.

Accessories, apart from specs which are covered later, should reflect both your scale and your bodyline. A medium size, stiff leather briefcase will look fantastic if you are a medium scale and angular man. If you're contoured, opt for a fabric that moves, such as suede or a softer leather.

Large scale

Fabrics should be the heaviest weights. Suiting about 14oz.

Patterns should be large and also reflect your bodyline, for instance a large check tie would look great on a large scale, angular man. Opt for large swirls or paisleys if you're contoured.

Accessories, apart from specs which are covered later, should reflect both your scale and your bodyline. A large briefcase will look fantastic on a large scale man. Choose stiff leather if you're angular and a softer leather if you're contoured.

Ties should have some width or your body will look bigger.

If you still don't understand the mechanics of scale or why you should bother, imagine this scenario – a very small business man carrying (or is that dragging) an extremely large briefcase. He probably thinks the case makes him look important, but in fact, the size differential gives the impression that he is even smaller and therefore less significant.

SHIRTS AND TIES

The most popular and safe choice for a formal shirt is a plain colour. Usually this is white followed by pale blue. A dark shirt is considered to be casual. The second choice is stripes, followed by checks. The narrower or smaller the pattern, the more formal it is.

The traditional way of wearing a shirt and tie is to have the shirt lighter than the suit and the tie darker than the shirt. A more contemporary look is to wear shirt and tie in very similar tones, with a suit that is only slightly darker. A very light tie on a dark shirt, which is also darker than a suit, looks like you belong to the Mafia and is to be avoided at all costs – unless you do belong to the Mafia, that is.

Your tie should just touch the belt or waistband of your trousers. Too short and you will look like a naughty schoolboy. Too long and it will look like a sporran. You should never wear a tie with a short sleeved shirt.

When tying a tie, make sure you balance the size of knot with the dimensions of the collar.

A Point collar looks better with a narrower four in hand knot.

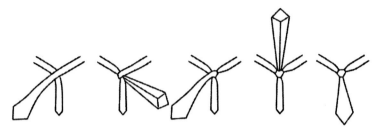

A Spread collar needs a Half-Windsor.

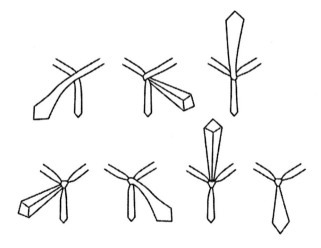

A big Italian collar needs a Double Windsor.

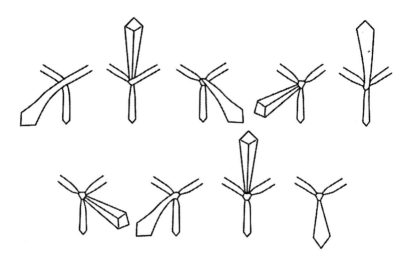

Shirt collars should fit correctly around the neck and should show about ½ - ¾ inch above your jacket. Cuffs should be loose enough to accommodate your watch but not so loose that your wrists dangle below.

COMBINING PATTERNS

Three solid colours together, as long as they don't clash, is a safe bet and can look sophisticated.

Two solids and one pattern is easy to wear well.

One solid and two patterns – leave this to the younger generation as it can look 'interesting' if not managed correctly.

Three patterns – completely eccentric!

ACT YOUR AGE

Nothing looks more ridiculous than a 50-year-old woman wearing a mini skirt, fish net tights and 4 inch stilettos. The same philosophy applies to men. Fashion is not just for the young *but* you do need to know what is and isn't appropriate. People respond readily to someone who is stylish and self aware, whatever their profession or economic status. Someone in their 40s trying to look like someone in their 20s, even if they are rich and respectable, will soon become the object of ridicule.

Here are some items that I find regularly in older men's wardrobes. If you have them, they need to be thrown out   NOW!

- Sweaters with patterns in bright colours á la Val Doonican
- Christmas or novelty sweaters
- Leather trousers
- Jeans – if you're over 45 be careful; they can age you
- Denim jackets – again denim can age you.
- Leather bomber jackets
- Tweed jackets with leather patches on the elbows
- Hawaiian shirts
- Coloured/patterned formal dinner shirts with matching cummerbund
- Tie-dye T-shirts
- T- shirts advertising a rock concert (or anything with a slogan or motif)
- White socks (unless they are used for sport)
- Coloured, patterned or novelty socks
- Tiny swimming shorts
- Tatty underwear
- Underwear that doesn't suit you – Y fronts or patterned boxers for instance
- Vests
- Cowboy Boots
- Moccasins
- Sandals with socks
- Novelty Ties (they are REALLY not funny)
- Anything you wore ten years ago

Clothes don't have to be terribly expensive or have a designer label to look fabulous. The main thing is to buy only items that fit you perfectly and that also enhance your natural body shape.

LET'S FACE IT

"There is no such thing as a plain face"
David Levine, Caricaturist

Your face is probably the most important part of your body. It's often the first thing we notice about someone, whether in a business meeting or across a crowded room.

You may look in the mirror and worry whether you have more wrinkles, bags under your eyes or spots or you may be like my husband and never look in the mirror at all!

Understanding the shape of your face and your features will help you to look more authentic. This, in turn, will enhance your natural good looks. You'll be able to choose hairstyles and spectacles that really do you justice. It will also affect how you wear your shirt and tie.

Exercise:

Using a mirror, look at your facial features.

Is your nose a) long and straight or is it b) small short or full?

Do your eyebrows a) sit straight or are they b) arched?

Are your eyes a) small or almond shaped or b) large and round?

Do you have a) visible cheekbones and planes within your face or are your cheeks b) soft and plump?

Are your lips a) thin and straight or b) plump and large?

Is your chin a) square or angular or is it b) soft or rounded?

Keep your mirror handy as you'll need this later.

If you answered mainly a to each of the questions, you have angular features. If you answered mainly b your features are contoured. You may remember we touched on these terms when looking at body shapes. Don't worry if your features are different to your body shape. It is possible to have a body that is one shape and a face that is another.

If you have long hair, push it behind your ears so that the outline of your face is visible. Starting at the top of your head, use both hands to trace the outline with your fingertips so you can really see its shape. Is it round, oval, square, rectangular? Do you have a more pronounced jawline? If so, is your face a diamond, a heart, a triangle or a pear?

On the whole, people with angular features will have a square or rectangular face. If the jaw is more pronounced, then it can be diamond or triangle. Contoured features normally reside in an oval, round, heart or pear shaped face.

If you're still not sure, take a look at the following descriptions:

The description of spectacle frames also applies to sunglasses. By the way, if you have a long nose, avoid a high metal bridge on your glasses. A solid, plastic frame, without nose pads will instantly shorten your nose.

OVAL

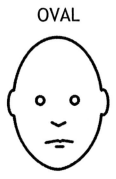

The face shape thought to be the most perfect and the one to aspire to!

Forehead is slightly wider than the chin.

Features are well balanced and proportioned.

Suits most hairstyles, spectacles and collars.

ROUND

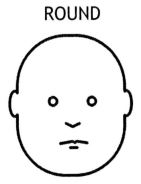

Similar in height and width.

Full cheeks and rounded jawline.

Need to make the face look longer and suits hairstyles with height or length.

A fringe is not advisable.

Spectacles should sit inside the outline of the face to narrow it. A thin bridge will lengthen the nose. Avoid round styles as you will look like an owl!

Avoid cutaway collars.

HEART

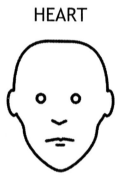

The forehead and cheekbones are wide. The jaw and chin are narrow.

Balance the face by adding width to the lower half.

Hair looks good if it's worn slightly longer, without a fringe.

A side or off centre parting can suit this face shape.

Spectacles, which have a coloured rim at the bottom and clear glass at the top look fantastic on this shape of face.

Cutaway collars look good but avoid long or pointed ones.

PEAR

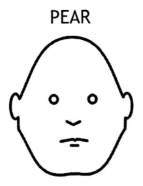

The widest point of the face is at ear level. The jaw is quite defined and the forehead narrow.

Need to make the forehead wider.

Hair should be kept close at the sides, have some height and weight on top (to balance the jawline) and be kept off the forehead. Avoid hair round the neck.

Spectacle frames should be heavier on the top than the bottom and be slightly rounded.

Longer collars and button down shirts are the most flattering.

SQUARE

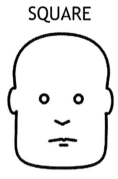

Straight sides, wide forehead and very square jawline.

Need to narrow and soften.

Avoid heavy fringes as these reduce the amount of face visible.

Suits hairstyles with height or length. A layered cut using gel looks great

Keep the sides cropped close to the head as fullness will add too much width.

An off centre parting may narrow the face.

Spectacles should be narrower than the face. High sides and a high bridge will add length.

Collars look better if longer. Avoid cutaways.

RECTANGLE

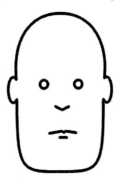

Longish face with straight sides and a wide forehead.

Need to balance the length by creating width.

Hair should be full to provide width.

A fringe (full or partial) will reduce length.

Men look best with short hair that lacks height.

Spectacles should be wider than the outline of the face. This creates a horizontal line which widens and shortens.

Wider shirt collars will add width. Avoid long collars.

DIAMOND

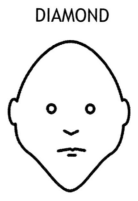

Cheeks are the widest point. Forehead and chin are narrower.

Need to widen both forehead and chin

Hair can be full at the forehead or the chin.

A side parting or side fringe will help disguise narrow forehead.

Hair should be cut close to the ears as this is the widest point

Specs should be narrower than the outline of the face.

Cutaway collars give the illusion of width.

TRIANGLE

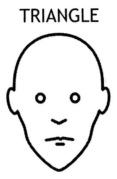

Face will taper to a narrow chin making the forehead look wide.

Needs to create width around chin area.

Hair should add visual width at the back of the head.

Spectacles should be narrower than the outline of the face. If possible, they should be wider on the bottom than the top.

Cutaway collars add width.

On the whole, general style principles apply just as they did to your body shape. If you have an angular face, think stiff fabrics around the neck, geometric shaped glasses and sharp haircuts. Contoured faces need more softness and look good with wavier hair, slightly curved frames and softer fabrics round the neck.

HAIR TODAY GONE TOMORROW

It's really important to choose an up to date style that suits you. My husband had a floppy type of hair style when I met him. Although his hair was in good condition, he has a square face and the style did nothing for him. He now sports a short spiky cut and it really has taken years off him.

Ponytails do not look cool if you're over 40. Even David Seaman has now seen sense and divested himself of it. If you normally use a barber, try a salon. I know it's scary, but a good hair stylist can really make a positive difference to the way you look.

What if you're losing your hair? It's actually simple – cut it as short as you can. You may not want to shave your entire head. The shape of your underlying skull is vital to the success of this look, but a short, well-cut hair style can still look sexy and appealing.

There are other options, of course. A toupee, or growing your hair longer on one side and sweeping it over like Arthur Scargill are alternatives. I think you know by now that these are not viable. Looking graceful and dignified no matter what your age is what this book is about. No-one will be fooled. You will still look like a man who is wearing a toupee or combing over his hair.

Luckily, greying hair can look distinguished as a man grows older, giving more authority, but if you really can't stand it, then visit a professional. Highlights and colour treatments are high maintenance. A stylist will be able to advise the correct shade for your skin tone. If you do it yourself, you are liable to go too dark or too auburn, a sure giveaway. Coloured hair can take years off you but, if it goes wrong, you can find you have become a figure of fun.

TO BEARD OR NOT TO BEARD?

Facial hair can make a big difference to the shape of your face and the way you look. A moustache can help to disguise a large area between the bottom of the nose and the top lip. A goatee beard can look "artistic" and a full beard "academic". Facial hair can be frowned upon in certain industries, and a full beard can sometimes be perceived as unprofessional. Whatever you decide, if you have facial hair, ensure it is well trimmed and tidy.

LOOKS GOOD ON YOU

The same thing goes for your specs. I've lost count of the number of men I've met wearing large, round, metal frames. These were fashionable in the 90's. What does this say about their ability to stay in touch with the times?

Find yourself a good optician who not only knows how to test your eyes but who understands face shapes, and how spectacles can enhance your features too.

Your face is important. It is uniquely yours. Make the most of it and it could be your biggest asset yet.

COLOUR YOUR LIFE

"Pink is not a colour, it's a state of mind"
unknown

It's always a safe bet to stick with solid colours in darker tones and clean lines for your basic wardrobe. Wearing the wrong colour though, may make you look less than your best.

Hundreds of years ago, man did not have names for all the colours we have today. Modern technology has produced a myriad of new shades for us to delight in.

One way of labelling, that has been with us from the start, is that of a warm shade (yellow based) and a cool shade (blue based). Also an awareness of the differences between dark and light and bright and soft will help. These characteristics are what image consultants base our colour analysis on today. By using specific coloured drapes, we can pick out colours which share the same characteristics as the complexion, thus making you look wonderful when you wear them.

This will be a do it yourself exercise and while it might not provide as in-depth advice as you'd get from a colour analysis it *will* help to eliminate those colours that really don't suit you while highlighting those that do.

One in four men are colour blind and one in seven cannot distinguish between different tones or shades of the same colour so ask your wife, mom, sister or girlfriend to help if you think you're one of them.

Exercise:

You'll need a mirror for this exercise. It's also useful to have someone with you as they can be more objective.

To check which colours suit you best, hold fabrics that are individually dark, light, cool (blue/pink based) and warm (yellow based) against your face. Record it on the chart below:

Very	In Between	Very
Dark/Deep		Light/Fair
Bright/Vivid/ Contrast		Muted/Soft/Subtle
Cool/pink/blue tones		Warm/gold/brown tones

Observe what happens to your skin.

Some colours may cast shadows giving a "grey" look around the jaw or under the eyes.

Warm colours on a cool skin may result in a jaundiced look.

Bright colours will suit you if you have bright eyes or a contrasting complexion (think Martin Kemp/Richard E Grant).

Soft, muted colours will suit those with less contrast between hair, eyes and skin (think Brad Pitt/Jamie Oliver).

Colours that are too bright can overwhelm and look garish – a good example of the clothes wearing you rather than the other way round.

Shades that are too muted can give the face a wishy-washy appearance with no real definition to the features.

Write down what has happened and use this for the basis of selecting colours in the future. If you looked good in dark and bright colours, choose these as soft and light colours probably will not suit you. If the warmer tones of yellow and cream suited you, odds are the cooler tones of blue and pink will not be flattering.

There are 4 main types of colouring. You may find that you weren't able to tick 3 boxes, so go with the two characteristics that were the strongest:

WINTER	AUTUMN	SUMMER	SPRING
Dark, Cool & Bright	Dark, Muted & Warm	Light, Cool & Muted	Light, Bright & Warm
Dark or grey hair Bright blue, hazel, brown or black eyes Skin can be fair to very dark. It may have a high contrast to the hair Look of high contrast or strength	Golden blonde, auburn or brown hair Soft shades of green, hazel or brown eyes Skin tone is soft, similar to eye colour with no real contrast and will have a sun kissed look or freckles Look of warmth or richness	Light to medium ash blonde, mousy or cool light red hair Pale blue, grey, green or hazel eyes Blue undertones to the skin show in a pinkiness which can be fair or medium Look of delicateness or, English rose	Golden blonde or warm light brunette/ red hair Bright shades of blue, green, hazel and brown Yellow undertones show as a sun kissed look on the skin, which will be fair. Look of lightness, and brightness

It may be helpful to think about the colours you will find during each of the seasons, as these will be the ones that best suit you:

Winter: Bold, dramatic landscapes, with white snow, black trees shed of their leafage, grey skies, deep red berries. This palette includes the bright, deep primary colours, except yellow, and the icy tones of very pale blue, green, pink, violet and white. You can wear suiting in black and charcoal well.

Autumn: Trees with leaves of all shades of gold, orange, green, yellow, red and brown give a good insight into the colours which suit this complexion. They are soft shades and not bright. Cream is a better choice than white. You will look better in chocolate brown or navy suiting. Olive green looks especially good.

Summer: Soft shades of pink, lavender, blue and lemon. All pastels look good on this complexion. Imagine the sun has faded the colours of the flowers in bloom so they are no longer bright but have muted tones. Off white is more suitable than a bright white. You will suit grey and a soft navy rather than black in tailored garments.

Spring: Flowers are emerging such as daffodils, and crocuses. Bright shades that have a yellowish tinge but are light rather than dark. Corals, light green and turquoise fit nicely into this palette. Ivory is a better choice than white, which is too cool. You will look good in pale linen colours, beige or brown, rather than black.

DRESSING TO CHANGE YOUR APPROACH

There are times in our lives when we can become anxious or nervous. It might be a presentation to the board, a blind date, meeting your girlfriend's mother for the first time and so on. At times like these we could all do with a little help, without hitting the gin bottle.

You may not be aware of it, but colour is a powerful medium when it comes to tackling everyday situations. You may even be wearing a colour which sends out a signal, albeit subconsciously. Pink, for instance, is thought to be the colour of love, so wearing it may be an attempt to surround ourselves with love or even attract love into our lives.

Think about situations that might cause anxiety in your life, or occasions when you need to be motivated. Using the following guide, discover how wearing a particular colour can help and assist you when you most need it. The colour does not have to apply to the entire outfit, sometimes just a splash will do the trick.

Red – Red has the longest wavelength, so we see it first (think traffic lights, brake lights and so on). It is stimulating and courageous. Wear it if you want to be noticed, powerful, assertive or strong. Politicians often wear a red tie when they have something important to say. The red imitates the colouring in the lips so you will automatically look at the mouth.

Orange – A mixture of yellow and red symbolising passion, abundance and fun. Beware though, unless you are deeply tanned, not many of us carry off this colour well. So wear as a complimentary or accent colour unless you want to be Tango'd!

Yellow – An emotional colour that governs extraversion, friendliness, creativity and optimism. It represents our personal power and how we feel about ourselves. A spot of yellow can go a long way to making you feel more confident. This colour looks better on people with darker skins, so beware of overdoing it.

Green – The least worn colour in the UK, perhaps because of its 'unlucky' connotations. Green signifies balance, compassion and understanding – think green for "go" as in traffic lights. A useful colour to wear if you have a difficult client, a confrontation or an apology to make! Also useful to enable balance within if you feel "out of sorts". Bright lime green suits very few people and can reflect back onto the face giving a green shadow around the jaw. Unless you want to look like an alien, choose a darker or softer alternative.

Blue – Governs speech, communication, creative expression and intellect. Wear it when presenting a speech or if you need a clear thought pattern. A serene and soothing colour, it mentally calms. Interestingly, Tony Blair and George W Bush both wore dark navy suits during the Iraq crisis. The message – trust us, we know what we are doing.

Purple – A spiritual colour which is also thought to represent authenticity, truth and luxury (Cadbury's Dairy Milk was perceived to be very expensive chocolate due to its purple wrapper). It has many links with royalty and the church due to its expensive price years ago. It can look good in a tie or as a pinstripe on a shirt.

Pink – Love and femininity. Yes, even macho men have a feminine side so you can still wear pink with pride. A soothing colour which radiates warmth and love.

Brown – Earthy and reliable, though can be construed as dull. Brown is warmer and softer than black and can look more flattering on warmer skins. For maximum impact, stick to darker shades. Wear if you want to elicit trust and openness.

Black – Everyone's favourite 'safe' bet. Exudes sophistication, efficiency, authority and security. Often worn as a slimming aid (though this does not work for everyone) it can drain and become serious. Wear with caution unless you know it suits you. Black suits should be restricted to funerals and other formal occasions.

White – White is a total reflection and represents purity. Can be perceived as hygienic and sterile which is why it's used in hospitals and clinics worldwide.

Grey – A neutral colour. Grey can have a dampening effect on other colours and can indicate a lack of confidence. However, charcoal grey is a great colour for suiting.

Your clothes can also have an effect when you need to modify your behaviour to get the best result.

Exercise:

First of all I'd like you to think about your own personality. Where would you sit on a scale of 1 – 10 with shy/accepting at 1 and authoritative/domineering at 10? Are there certain circumstances when it would be beneficial to move up or down the scale to appear more or less demanding?

The way you put your clothes together can help you to achieve this.

One of my clients is a manager of a sales team. He is expected to get great results and, on the whole, he achieves this. However, he realised that many of the team seemed to be in awe of him and rarely did any of them call him for help. Even during team meetings he felt that he was doing all the talking and the input from his team was minimal.

We looked at his style of dress. He was wearing a charcoal grey, well-tailored suit, white crisp cotton shirt and a deep red tie. He looked fabulous *but* without knowing it, his adopted style was that of an authoritarian.

I suggested he toned down the colours so there would be less contrast between them. A paler grey suit with blue shirt and blue tie, for instance. As a result, he still looked like a smart businessman *but* now he appeared to be more approachable. The result – his staff opened up more to him as they felt less intimidated.

Here are some tips that will help you to adapt and connect more effectively with people:

1. Authority is gained by wearing clothes with maximum contrast: black and white, dark brown and cream, navy and palest blue.

2. A softer image is gained by dressing in tones and shades of a single colour: brown or green trousers and slightly lighter shade for the upper body.

3. Plain, bold colour is authoritative.

4. Introduce pattern or design for a softer look, for instance a paisley tie with a striped shirt.

5. The larger the stripe or check in a shirt the more casual it appears.

6. A jacket that compliments, but doesn't exactly match your trousers will appear less authoritative. A jacket worn with a T-shirt or a polo shirt will appear less formal than a shirt and tie.

7. Fabrics that are stiff and starchy will appear more authoritative than those that have more fluidity and drape. The same applies to garments with lots of fitted tailoring (authority) and less structure (approachable).

8. Red and/or black can look severe. Pastels will appear less so.

9. A button down collar in a softer fabric will look less authoritative than a stiff cutaway.

10. Hairstyles that are severe will give an impression of power. The same applies to your spectacles. Black rimmed glasses are more authoritative than rimless ones.

SMART CASUAL – THE CONUNDRUM EXPLAINED

"There are times when you have to choose between being human and having good taste"
Bertolt Brecht

What is smart casual exactly? This is such a tough one to answer and I get asked it all the time. The words 'smart' and 'casual' seem to have opposite meanings, so it's easy to see why people get confused.

I'm going to put this into the context of business and the 'dress down Friday' or off-site team meetings. If you want to be casual in your leisure hours, you'll be looking at sweaters, casual shirts, T-shirts, cargo pants, cords, shorts and a casual jacket, suited to your particular body shape of course.

First of all it's never a good idea to split your business suit. Your suit jacket will always look like a business suit jacket and the same with the trousers. These days, if you're young, you can get away with wearing a business suit with a polo shirt, T- shirt or fine knit. If you're older, I'd stay clear and wear your suit with the traditional shirt and tie.

Be cautious of wearing linen or silk mixes, as they can crease/shine and look unkempt.

A casual business jacket, teamed with an open neck polo shirt and business casual trousers can look professional and casual at the same time. A plain cashmere sweater can also look good as long as you don't have a beer belly. Layering a T-shirt or shirt, with a thin V-neck sweater and a coordinating colour jacket can look great if you're slim. If you are underweight, you can use this layering method as a way to look bigger. It certainly works better than wearing bulky sweaters that will drown you.

Button down collars on your shirts are less formal than cutaway, as they are the only shirt which can be successfully worn without a tie. Steer clear of a white shirt or one with a contrasting collar (white collar with blue stripes on the main garment). Instead, wear a jacket and shirt in toning shades for a more approachable look. My husband wears a lightweight suit in olive green, with a soft shirt in a slightly deeper shade really successfully. Suede shoes and a brown belt complete the look. If he wants to look slightly more formal, he adds a coordinating patterned tie.

Shirts worn outside your trousers are intended for your leisure activities, rather than work. It can look very scruffy on an older man, especially if it has a large, bold pattern. If you're unsure how to wear your shirt correctly then follow this rule of thumb: shirts with tails should be worn inside your trousers, those with straight hems can be worn outside.

Jeans should be avoided in the workplace, as should cargo pants and any style with a drawstring. Choose moleskin trousers, chinos, gabardine, cotton drill, cords or wool worsted as a safer option.

Make sure that your footwear is also less formal. Choose suede as an alternative to leather, wear loafers, slip-ons or half boots rather than oxford brogues. Perhaps look to brown rather than black, as long as it coordinates with the rest of your outfit. Leave the trainers for your sporting activities.

Belts too, can be less formal but should still match the colour of your shoes.

DRESSING FOR THE OCCASION

*"If you haven't got any socks,
you can't pull them up"*
Jeffrey Barnard

There are certain situations where dressing appropriately is vital. Funerals, weddings, job interviews, court appearances and formal dinners fit into this category. Wearing incorrect attire is usually as a result of the following:

- You've made a faux pas and you feel ridiculous and embarrassed.

- You've deliberately dressed in your own style, knowing that it's inappropriate, but you don't care.

In both cases, you will stand out like a sore thumb and you'll definitely be noticed – even if it's for the wrong reasons.

The first instance is often a case of mis-judgement or not taking the time to ask for guidelines. It can be painful. If you wanted to make a good impression, you may find yourself on the outside, keeping your head down throughout the proceedings. Often a hard lesson to learn if the occasion was important to your career or relationship.

The second is a case of arrogance whichever way you look at it.

On certain occasions, following a dress code is a mark of respect to the rest of the attendees. Imagine you have booked a meal at a top class, expensive and exclusive restaurant for you and your partner, perhaps for a very special occasion. How would you feel if you were served by a waiter/waitress dressed in shabby clothes with body piercings and tattoos? Severely let down and unimpressed I would think.

So why would you dress in jeans for a formal dinner, a funeral or a job interview in the city? Unless there are specific instructions to wear whatever you wish, always check beforehand. If it's impossible for you to comply, then check that it's OK with the organisers first. Remember, the impression you make may have a lasting effect on someone who has influence in the future.

FORMAL DINNERS

Black tie is the utmost in elegance and, as every woman will tell you, all men (with no exceptions) look handsome in this type of dress.

There are a number of different styles of dinner jacket for you to choose from:

The Shawl Collar. This has a smooth lapel with no notched V. Personally, it's not my favourite but it does have a kind of relaxed appeal.

Peaked Lapels. This is a very wide and extremely sharp lapelled jacket. Suitable only for angular bodies.

Notched Lapels. This is the most common as it resembles a normal suit jacket. Easier to wear but without the panache of the peaked lapel.

Double or single breasted? We've looked at these style options previously. Single breasted will always get my vote. Double breasted can look dated and should only be worn by the tall and slim.

White or Ivory Tuxedo. Can look extremely elegant if you have the right colouring and want to stand out from the crowd.

You can wear braces and a waistcoat if you have a large stomach instead of the traditional cummerbund. The latter may emphasise a large waist due to its horizontal nature.

Shirts should be white, preferably with a double cuff that can accommodate your cufflinks. Remember that your face shape will determine the type of collar that best suits it. A stiff winged collar will not flatter you if you have a round or chubby face. Choose a turn down collar instead. Also remember your scale. If you are large scale, you will need a wider bow tie.

Shoes should be dress shoes, usually in black patent leather and highly polished.

OTHER BUSINESS OCCASIONS

Casual – no tie required but you need to dress smartly. A jacket or suit is optional.

Semi Formal – Dark suit and black shoes

Black Tie Optional – A tuxedo is required. A black suit will suffice.

White Tie – A highly formal affair. Requires a tailcoat, white tie and white cummerbund or waistcoat.

FUNERAL

Unless you have specific instructions not to wear it, black is the order of the day here. In fact, black suits were traditionally only worn at funerals. Dark, chargoal grey is for the office.

JOB INTERVIEW

Often we're under the illusion that gaining promotion or getting a new job is all about our ability to do the job well. In other words, how well qualified we are.

Robert Half's research on promotional prospects underlines how vital it is to have the correct image. Only 10% of your potential for success is concerned with actually doing the job well. Image accounts for a substantial 30% and networking and personal promotion a massive 60%.

You would always research the company you hope to work for, but it is essential to also research their dress code and culture. Advertising and PR agencies, for instance, may not put the same emphasis on a suit and tie as a finance company or a bank.

Other touches that may help the process are: a good quality pen, a stylish leather briefcase (remember scale), diary/palm pilot and/or laptop and a non-digital watch with a metal or leather strap (keep sports watches for sporting activities) and modern spectacles (if needed). Don't flaunt jewellery or ostentatious watches and don't over do the aftershave. Most importantly – switch off your mobile.

COURT APPEARANCE

What can I say? Just make sure you look groomed and respectable. That means your business suit, freshly pressed shirt, tie and polished shoes. Ditch the jewellery, clean your fingernails, tidy your hair and try not to smoke.

FIRST DATE

As with the job interview, you need to do some research. What do you know about her? How old is she? What does she like doing? Where are you going to meet? This is the key criteria on which to base your decision on what to wear. Once that's decided, you can then dress appropriately, using the guidelines in this book. Remember, the first impression you make will have a massive impact. Once you've got through that, you can use your charm and listening skills to wow her.

WHAT YOUR BEST FRIEND
WON'T TELL YOU

"What is elegance? Soap and water!"
Cecil Beaton, Photographer

Every Sunday morning, I can look down the street and see all my male neighbours diligently waxing and polishing their pride possession – their car. The care they take is unbelievable. They stand back and admire their handiwork, with an expression of rapture on their faces. Each one of them spends hours every week on this ritual and none seem to mind. How is it then that the same amount of time spent on the car is not spent when polishing up their *own* appearance?

Most men will instantly notice the smallest scratch on their car's paintwork, so how do they not notice the bush of hair escaping from their nostrils? You will wax, polish and buff your car to gleaming perfection, but will not spend even 10 seconds moisturising your own bodywork.

My husband is a car dealer, so I know what I'm talking about. He is also in his late 50s and a bit of a 'macho' man. However, in the last couple of years, he has seen the difference that grooming can make. He has his daily routine, which takes him a minimal amount of time, and sticks to it. The pay back includes the compliments he gets about how young he looks, the fuss that the 'John Lewis girls' make when he purchases new products, a younger wife who thinks he looks sexy, and clients who regard him as a true professional.

If you don't like the word 'vain' then use 'self-respect' instead. It boils down to the same thing. It is healthy to want to care for yourself.

You may of course want to be pro-active in your grooming routine but are confused by the array of products on the shelves. This chapter will simplify the processes and the jargon, so you can gleam and shine, just like your car.

THE ESSENTIALS

The following products should appear in your bathroom cabinet.

If you're unsure of what some of these items are relax, all will be explained as you work through the chapter. You can ask for help and advice from the cosmetic counters of any large department store, but if this is too scary, try your local supermarket. Brands like Nivea have a great range of men's products which you can buy along with your weekly food shopping.

Item	Why?	Y/N
Facial Cleanser	Soap is too harsh to clean the face and strips the skin of moisture	
Skin Toner	Use with cotton wool to close pores after cleansing, especially if you have oily skin	
Moisturiser SP15	Softens the skin, reduces wrinkles and can protect from sun damage	
Facial Exfoliator	Removes dead skin cells and helps prevent in growing hairs - use prior to shaving	
Shaving Cream	Wraps the hair making it easier to shave and less likely to get shaving rash/burn or	

	cuts	
Razor	A wet shave is better than a dry one as it gets closer to the root of the hair	
Shampoo	Specifically selected for your hair type, especially if you have dandruff or greasy hair	
Conditioner	Moisturises the hair to make it shiny and healthy looking and easier to comb	
Hair styling products	To style and groom your hair	
Deodorant	To prevent underarm odour	
Nose Hair Trimmer	Essential if you're over 30 to get rid of that bush in your nose and ears	
Eyebrow Tweezers	To keep unruly eyebrows at bay	

Nail Clippers	Easier to use than nail scissors. To maintain well kept hands and feet	
Hair Comb	To maintain neat and tidy hair throughout the day	
Toothbrush (preferably battery)Toothpaste and Dental Floss	Teeth should be brushed at least twice a day and flossed every night, especially if you smoke Change your toothbrush every 2 months	
Sun Tan Protection SP15 minimum	Skin cancer is growing. It makes sense to protect against it – if you work outdoors, this is absolutely essential	
Body Shampoo/ Washing Cream	Kinder and milder than soap for your body. Keeps the skin moisturised	

These are the absolute basics. If it reads like a foreign language, read on for explanations.

FACING UP TO IT

Women are bombarded with a myriad of new skin products every single day of their lives. Luckily, for you, life can be simpler. The premise is this: your skin is your armour against the outside elements. It also reflects whether or not you are healthy or ill. If you look after it, it will return the compliment by looking vibrant, radiant and youthful and be in a better position to protect.

To prevent against leathery, ageing skin or a dull, tired complexion you need to drink water. Lots of it. Preferably 2 litres a day. Unfortunately, beer doesn't count, neither does tea or coffee. Try to sip a little throughout the day, rather than drinking a pint in one sitting. You'll notice an improvement very quickly. As water will fill you up, this is also a good way to shed extra pounds if you need to.

SKIN TYPES

There are 3 main skin types, as follows:

Skin Type	Characteristics	Products
Normal	You probably won't have many problems. Perhaps the odd spot or a patch of dry skin occasionally.	Foaming cleanser SP15 Moisturiser
Oily	Prone to spots. Large open pores.	Gentle Cleanser Toner (to close pores) Oil Free Moisturiser Clear Pore Strip (Nivea) to remove blackheads around the nose
Dry	Tightness after washing and dry patches on the face. Lines and wrinkles. Possible ruddy complexion.	Gentle/cream cleanser Cream moisturiser SP15 for day Rich moisturiser for night

There is also a Combination skin type, which as the name suggests, combines oily and dry. If you have this, you will find the oiliness on the T-zone. This is the panel that runs across your forehead and down your nose to your chin (hence the name). You will need to use a combination of products as detailed above or look to the makeup counters for specific products.

The products detailed in the chart should be used every day, both morning and night, for best results. Once you get used to it, you'll wonder how you ever managed with a plain old bar of soap.

A CLOSE SHAVE?

Exfoliators are tiny granules, which when rubbed onto wet skin, remove the top layer of dead cells from your face. This top layer can build up over time making the skin look lifeless and dull. Regular exfoliation will bring back radiance to your complexion. It can also improve the quality of your shave and helps prevent razor burn and ingrowing hairs.

Exfoliate after cleansing, so your face is slightly damp. Rub the granules/cream gently over the face and then rinse off with warm water. This is then the time to shave. Once you have finished shaving, pat the face dry and use your toner and/or moisturiser.

SHAVING FOR PERFECT RESULTS

You can shave in the shower if you want to save time, but I still think time taken using a mirror has better results as you can see what you're doing. You don't want to leave the house with stray hairs on top of your lip do you?

Once you have exfoliated, the heat of the warm water in the shower or the basin will have opened up your hair follicles, allowing your beard to be removed with less risk of injury.

Work in your shaving cream using your fingers, or use a shaving brush if you prefer. Using a razor that has a moveable head, follow the natural grain of your hairs. Usually this means down the face rather than up. Dip the razor into water to unclog and to maintain a smooth cut. If you still have persistent stubble, shave again but across the grain this time.

Disposable razors/razor blades should be discarded immediately if they feel like they are pulling rather than cutting.

If you are very dark and/or grow hair throughout the day, take a battery operated razor with you. Have a quick buzz before meeting clients to keep your appearance professional.

There are specialist pre shaving oils on the market. My husband loves his as it makes his skin very smooth before shaving. It's your choice whether or not you want to make an extra purchase but they can be useful if you have dry skin.

AFTER SHAVE

Moisturise after shaving and then splash with your favourite scent. Aftershave lotions should not burn or sting, so if yours does, then be sensible and daub behind the ears instead.

NOSE AND EARS

While we're on the subject of facial hair, let's get to grips with the less attractive type. Nose hairs and ear hairs are a real turn off, yet most men don't seem to even notice their existence.

My husband was case in point, but he soon got the message when I started leaving 'GROOMING DAY!' post-it notes on the bathroom door. It was hard work, but the results were worth it. I'm hoping you'll just take this on board and get on with it – PLEASE!

You will need to invest in a battery operated nose clipper. The alternative is to snip with scissors or use eyebrow tweezers. As there are many nerve endings in your nose, you will probably be a masochist if you prefer the latter. The whole job will take less than 5 minutes, both nose and ears. Schedule it in every week. It can be so off putting for those people who need to look at you every day. You'll find they are concentrating more on your nose hair than what you are actually saying. Not a good state of affairs to be in.

Eyebrows. Notice the plural. You have two eyes and two eyebrows. A monobrow, one that continues to grow in the area between your brows, is not attractive and it will need to be dealt with. If you're too scared to get the tweezers out, ask a beautician to wax. It's probably quicker and less painful. Both waxing and tweezing will eventually weaken the hair follicles so they will grow back less quickly.

As you age, your eyebrow hairs will want to go their own sweet way. Individual hairs that stick out from the main brow will need to be removed with tweezers. Stretch the skin tightly between two fingers. Using your other hand, grab the offending hair with the tweezers and yank towards your ears. Don't be a baby. It really doesn't hurt... that much.

You may also need to tidy any hairs that grow too far down the outer edges of your eyes. These can make you look tired, as they pull the eyes downwards.

If your eyebrow hairs are too long – another sign of age – trim them with scissors. If you're unsure, or your hand is unsteady, ask your hairdresser or a professional to do it for you.

Never shave eyebrow hair. It'll just encourage more growth.

BODY HAIR

The odd chest hair is not going to cause any great problems. If, however, you have hair that protrudes into your collar area or hair that covers the back of your shoulders, you may need to do something about it.

You can try waxing or using a depilatory cream at home. Both methods are simple to use but waxing may be painful. A depilatory cream will involve smoothing it on, waiting for a few minutes and then showering it off. The effect usually lasts about 1 month. It can also be used on underarm hair. Waxing may be best left to a professional.

Ridding yourself of underarm hair, as women do, will allow your deodorant to work better. If it hasn't got all that hair to fight, it will be more effective. If you don't already use a deodorant, please put it on your shopping list now. Many men are oblivious to their own body odour. Stale sweat is probably one of the most obnoxious smells around, and can cause embarrassment to colleague and friends. It's very difficult to actually tell someone that they smell bad. So make sure you never put yourself in this position.

HAIR PRODUCTS

There are *so* many products on the market, you'd be forgiven for being confused and walking away. The most suitable product for you will depend mainly on the hairstyle you have and also the effect you are trying to create.

I've listed 3 of the main products below. There are many more but I don't want to confuse the issue.

1. Styling Gel: Goes on wet and stays looking wet. Great for thick or curly hair. Rub through fingers and apply to hair, scrunching it into the style you require.

2. Sculpting Lotion: Thinner than gel and great for very short hair or wavy styles. Adds firmness, without looking stiff. A good option for thinning hair. It can be applied to wet hair, which will remain looking wet, or you can leave it for a few minutes and ruffle your fingers through your dry hair to make it look more natural.

3. Wax: This is for top duty hold so is good for longer, textured styles as well as short. Use if your hair is thick but it will be too heavy for thin hair. Adds gloss, shine

and manageability to the hair. Pomade is a similar product. With both products it's best to warm it in your hands before applying to dry hair. Not only will less go a longer way but it helps malleability.

HANDS AND FEET

To me there is nothing better than seeing a man with well tended hands. Unfortunately, they are few and far between. At worst, fingernails should be kept short and clean but a full manicure shouldn't go amiss once in a while. It will cost you about £10 and you'll be amazed at the difference. No – you won't have nail varnish applied, you'll just discover a beautiful set of fingernails and smooth, unblemished hands.

Feet can be a problem for most men, especially the hard, dry skin around the heels. If this applies to you, make a regular appointment with a chiropodist. They can rid you of yellowing skin, corns and callouses, and trim your toenails to perfection. You can, of course, use a pumice stone when showering or a foot cream manufactured for this purpose.

SMILE PLEASE

Americans call yellowish, crooked teeth "British Teeth". I wonder why? They go to great lengths to get a smashing set of pearly white gnashers. You will frequently see teenagers wearing braces to straighten their teeth. Cosmetic dentistry, such as teeth whitening is big business over the pond.

It may be too late for the braces but keeping your teeth in good condition is a must. Regular trips to your dentist and hygienist will ensure your teeth stay in tip top condition. If you leave it too long, you are putting yourself at greater risk of gum disease, bad breath and a yellowing smile. Not very attractive! Just do it.

YOUR BODY IS YOUR TEMPLE

Being pampered is not the exclusive domain of the female. If you've never tried it before, go and relax with a facial or an aromatherapy massage. Until you've succumbed, you won't know what you're missing. You deserve some relaxation time and, as a bonus, you'll look even more handsome.

WHO ARE YOU?

"Chic is a personal style that comes off with integrity"
Bernie Ozer

DRESSING AUTHENTICALLY

Now we get down to the real nitty gritty. You've established your overall body and face shape, the colours that best suit you, how to disguise any figure challenges, your grooming schedule and how to behave in public! Well done for getting this far.

But all of that counts for nothing if you don't feel comfortable with the overall result. Clothes should be an extension of your personality not a suit of armour or a mask. Dressing in a way that is authentic is absolutely vital to your levels of confidence and your ultimate success.

A client of mine works in an office environment where casual dress is the order of the day. He is in his late 40s, and a fairly shy and reserved man. He hates the idea of working in what he considers to be his 'leisure wear'. He has boundaries in his life and his clothes help define them. To him wearing casual clothes to the office would be as alien as wearing a suit to go the gym. He also realises that he needs to fit in and be part of the team. Between us, we've managed to create a look that fits in with his corporate lifestyle but also expresses his own unique personality. Instead of wearing casual clothes from top to toe, he wears chinos with a polo shirt and jacket and smart shoes. He feels professional, which is important for him to do his job effectively, but also looks quite casual in comparison to his fully suited look. His work/life boundaries are still in place, he fits in with the team and company culture and he feels proud of his appearance. Guess what? He is highly successful. Because he looks and feels confident, he commands the respect of his colleagues and his clients. All this is great news for the company's bottom line and his own promotional prospects.

There are some garments that scream out a message as soon as you see them. I'm thinking of novelty ties for example. While the wearer may think they are fun to wear, I can assure you that the rest of us do not! So be authentic but also remember the environment in which you work.

Exercise:

Think about the words you would use to describe yourself. Make a list and then narrow it down to 2 or 3 key adjectives.

Look at your style of dress. Does it fully express the words you've just used about yourself? If not, why not?

What can you do to dress in a more authentic manner?

Ask someone you trust to describe you. Are their descriptors the same as yours? If not, ask them why they see you differently. Does your style have anything to do with it? Are your clothes giving out the wrong impression?

What changes (if any) do you need to make?

As the Greek Philosopher, Epicetus once said "Know first who you are and then adorn yourself accordingly"

THE BARE ESSENTIALS

"A gossip is one who talks to you about others; a bore is one who talks to you about himself; and a brilliant conversationalist is one who talks to you about yourself"
Les Levine, Artist

This chapter is all about the interactive you. By now, you should know how to dress to impress and create the impact you need. But every day we need to interact with others, both socially and in a business capacity. How well you do will depend on your level of social skills and your knowledge of etiquette. The guidelines below may seem obvious but you'd be surprised how many men simply do not follow them correctly. Let them help you maintain your credibility and build your reputation as a charming gentleman.

PLEASED TO MEET YOU

The first thing we do when we meet someone for the first time is shake their hand. But how many of you

SUE DONNELLY

actually know whether or not your handshake is effective?

A limp-wristed handshake gives an impression of weakness or a damp squid.

One that only touches the tips of the fingers is perceived as timid. If a man does this when greeting a woman, it could be misconstrued as insulting i.e. you're not equal to me so I won't shake your whole hand.

A handshake that is too strong will not only hurt the receiver's fingers but can come across as aggressive or arrogant.

Pumping someone's hand is not necessary either - you may come across as an over-eager puppy.

Covering someone's hand with your other hand can appear patronising. Although it is often meant to be a friendly, warm gesture it can convey the impression of superiority. Politicians often do this to convey who's the boss.

Wet palms can be a real issue if you're tense or anxious. Rather than wiping on your jacket, spray with an antiperspirant before you meet. Keep one in your car if this is a regular occurrence for you or use wet wipes. If that's not feasible, run your wrists under the

88

cold water tap (and then dry them) before the meeting takes place.

If you haven't done so before, please take the time to ask someone for feedback on your handshake. It sounds crazy but the wrong type of handshake can give out the wrong signals right from the start. The correct handshake should meet web to web and be firm but not painful! And don't forget to make eye contact and smile. Looking away can appear shifty.

"DAAH-LING..."

In certain environments, kissing has replaced the handshake as the usual form of greeting. This especially prevalent in a female or creativity biased business arena.

When kissing, you should just make contact with each cheek *and that's all*. It is not an excuse for a slobber, a grope or a snog.

Kissing a woman's hand was common 20 years ago because it was not the done thing to shake a woman's hand. Most women today would find this gesture quite off putting unless done correctly – firmly, and definitely not to be lingered over. In a business context, most women would say that this type of gesture would not be welcome, especially if meeting for the first time.

How many kisses? This depends on the culture. Americans are single kissers, as are some Brits. The French are double kissers and Swiss, Dutch and Belgians are triple kissers. Follow the lead of your host if unsure.

ROUND THE WORLD IN 80 DAYS

Many business people now travel around the world. It is essential to acquire knowledge of the cultural differences surrounding global greetings. A weak handshake is considered to be ineffective in the western world but is common practice in the East. A whole book could be written on this subject so all I'll say is do your research in advance.

GROOMING

Anyone who owns a horse or a long haired cat or dog will understand the importance of grooming. A well-kept, glossy coat and clean claws can completely transform an animal from a straggly, unkempt one into a first class example of the species.

Most of us realise, at some level, that we need to look presentable when meeting other people. The essentials including a daily shower, washing hair, brushing, wearing clean, pressed clothes are mandatory, so I won't waste time mentioning them. Instead, I will reiterate some of the basics so that you get the message loud and clear.

A designer outfit will not make up for dirty fingernails.

Facial hair, such as a full beard, can be frowned upon in some corporate organisations. Modern companies, advertising agencies for instance, have a more relaxed attitude. If you're likely to acquire a shadow during the day, keep a battery powered shaver with you.

Nasal hairs – I've lost count of the number of times I've been riveted to a senior executive's nose rather than to what he is saying. *Please*, check in a mirror every day and remove any strays. This also applies to bushy hair growth in the ears and in the eyebrows. Bushy stray hair is also very ageing!

Don't overdo the aftershave. It can overpower rather than seduce.

Is your suit past its sell by date? Shiny material, scruffy shoes and a bobbled tie screams 'not bothered'.

Are you up to date? This does not necessarily mean trendy, but outdated clothes create an image that the wearer is not keeping up with current thinking. This applies to spectacles and briefcases, as well as clothing.

Keep jewellery to a minimum. A watch and wedding ring only. Bracelets, earrings and necklaces, especially on older men, can be perceived as 'Del Boy'. If you must wear a necklace, keep it hidden under your shirt.

Shoes should be polished, shirts pressed and clean. Ties should touch the waistband of your trousers and be appropriately knotted for the type of shirt you're wearing.

If you wear a pocket handkerchief, it should be a similar colour to your tie but not made from the same fabric.

BODY LANGUAGE

Whether or not we are aware of it, people are reading us all the time. Great fitting clothes and a professional image will go along way to making the right first impression but what you wear isn't the whole solution.

The way your body responds is crucial to appearing credible and authentic. If you say one thing but your body language says something else, it's the body language we'll believe.

Most of us have never been trained to read body language but actually *all* of us are experts. For instance, if you are speaking to someone who is lazing in their chair, arms behind their head and not making eye contact, you will make a judgement dependent on the situation. You may feel that he is arrogant and rude, especially if you've not met before. Alternatively, this may be someone's way of thinking about an answer to your question and he is just acting in a relaxed manner.

A first impression is like a filter. Psychological evidence shows that we put a lot of weight on initial information when evaluating someone. We all like to think we are a good judge of character – "I knew I couldn't trust him from the moment I met him". Later evidence may prove that your initial reaction was incorrect, but it is your first response that influences how you process information about that person from that point on. It's important, therefore, to ensure the first impression you make is a favourable one.

INFLUENCING TRIANGLE

The correct posture when you meet someone should be relaxed but showing energy and enthusiasm. Imagine a triangle with your head at its apex and both shoulders as the other points. This is called the Influencing Triangle and all your energy radiates from here. Slouching causes the energy to flow downwards instead of towards your companion. This is especially important for men as a badly fitting tie, shirt collar or jacket will instantly dilute the impact.

WHAT A POSER!

Crossing the arms across the chest implies a closed mind while hands on hips signifies aggression and potential confrontation.

Hands clasped behind the back may suggest: politely authoritative; snobbish; don't want to get my hands dirty.

Hands clasped in front over the groin area is seen as a very defensive posture – think of free kicks in the penalty box during a football match.

Legs crossed while standing implies a lack of confidence – or perhaps a need to visit the little boys room.

Edging away from the speaker displays arrogance or nervousness and an urge to avoid direct communication.

Lack of eye contact implies that you are shifty and not to be trusted.

FACIAL EXPRESSIONS

Is your expression open and receptive? Are you smiling? Are your brows open? Do you look interested? Are you making eye contact when you converse? Do you appear to be listening?

If your head is down, you are frowning, and/or your lips are pursed you may just be concentrating but, unfortunately, it can be interpreted as unreceptive and hostile.

The importance of congruence is paramount. If you're breaking some bad news it would be suicidal to smile and employ open handed gestures. So think tall, act positive, pay attention to your companion and you'll be a great success.

So you're groomed, listening attentively and radiating positive energy. Wonderful. Now it's your turn to speak. Your voice and what you say can make or break you, so here are some tips.

WHAT DID YOU SAY?

Are you audible so you can be clearly heard? Are your pitch and tone enthusiastic and modular?

Stress can tighten the back of the throat so we tend to speak in a higher vocal range (even squeak if we're really scared) and much faster than normal.

Accents can dominate someone's speech but luckily are far more acceptable these days than the traditional BBC voice of the past.

If you speak breathily, your messages may be conveyed as lacking depth or gravitas.

Swallowing your words at the end of a sentence, so they are not clear, can lead the listener to think you're hiding something.

If you have an important speech to make or you are nervous, it makes sense to exercise the voice. Sing a long to the radio or talk to yourself if necessary. Remember to pause for effect and that silence isn't necessarily a bad thing. It will always appear longer to you than it will to your audience.

SMALL TALK

Psychologists have proved that attractiveness, emotional expression and social skills all contribute to likeability. However, your attractiveness is the smallest contributing factor. Charm and social skills are the keys to successful communication and rapport.

Small talk is often thought to be the province of women. Men are more often concerned about what they are going to say and so get down to business immediately. This can appear extremely curt.

Enthusiasm is vital. This is often the main differentiator between you and your competitors. Elevate the mood by smiling and drawing attention to any positive or humorous aspects of the situation.

Find a connection. It may be detective novels or how the England cricket team is doing. It's easier to forge a bond with someone if you have shared interests.

Be curious. People like to talk about themselves. Show interest in them by asking questions.

Listen – you were born with one mouth and two ears. It's wise to use them in that ratio. Women adore a good listener, so make it a priority if it's a date you're after. Business relationships will also flourish if you've really listened to a client's needs and responded accordingly.

Last but not least. Do you have any distracting habits? You'll probably be the last to know even if you do. Please ask someone you trust. Research has proved that while someone you've met may not remember your name, or what you spoke about, they will definitely remember your distracting habits, several months later!

Consider the impact of your own personal image. For best results, ask a trusted friend to also complete on your behalf. Compare answers.

	An asset	Needs work
How You Look		
Clothes		
Accessories		
Grooming		
Hair		
How You Sound		
Voice		
Tone		
How You Act		
Handshake		
Eye Contact		
Posture		

Facial Expression		
Distracting Habits?		
How You Interact		
Social Skills		
Etiquette & Manners		
How You Are Perceived		
Enthusiasm		
Energy		
Positive Attitude		

PARETO IN YOUR WARDROBE

*"All that is not eternal is
eternally out of date"*
C S Lewis

In 1906, Italian economist Vilfredo Pareto noticed that twenty percent of the people owned eighty percent of the wealth. He created a mathematical formula to describe this unequal distribution which is now known as the Pareto' Principle (or 80/20 Rule). Essentially the formula states that twenty percent of your effort achieves eighty percent of your results.

Believe it or not, the same principle can apply to your wardrobe. If your wardrobe looks anything like some of my clients', I'd place a bet that you wear twenty percent of your clothes, eighty percent of the time. While it's always great to have choice, think how much that eighty percent is costing you.

Exercise:

To find out if your wardrobe is working for you, do the following exercise.

Take a piece of paper and draw two circles.

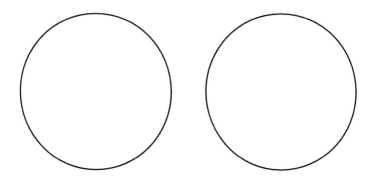

Using the circle as a pi chart, divide it into sections proportionate to the different areas of your life (excluding sleeping time). For instance, 40% may be work, 25% golf, 15% socialising, 10% gardening, 10% watching TV and so on.

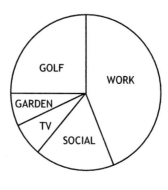

In the second circle, do the same thing with the clothes you own. For example, 20% of your clothes are suits, 25% are football shirts and so on.

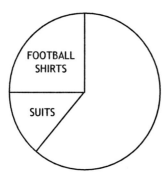

Now compare the results. Do they marry up or has one area totally dominated your wardrobe? Ask yourself why that might be. What are you hanging onto? What are you trying to avoid? If it does match up, then well done, you've got it just right.

The following is a guide to building a working man's wardrobe:

Need a suit every day	Don't need a suit every day
4-5 suits – mixture of dark colours and mid tones.	2-3 suits – mixture of dark colours and mid tones.
10-12 shirts – plain, fine striped, fine checked.	2 jackets
10-15 ties – this is your personal statement. Have enough to create different moods BUT no novelty ones.	3 pairs of trousers – to coordinate with the jackets. Never split suit jackets and trousers.
2 pairs shoes – wear on alternate days.	10-12 shirts – plain, fine striped, fine checked or a mix of shirts and polo shirts if the work environment is more casual.
10-12 pairs socks – to match shoes or suit colour.	8-10 ties – this is your personal statement. Have enough to create different moods BUT no novelty ones.
1-2 belts or braces – must always match shoes. Belts should be 1-1¼ inches wide with discreet buckles.	2 pairs shoes – wear on alternate days.
1 briefcase – according to scale and body shape.	10-12 pairs socks – to match shoes or suit colour
1 overcoat	

1 raincoat	1-2 belts or braces- must always match shoes. Belts should be 1-1¼ inches wide with discreet buckles
1 pair gloves - leather	
1 scarf - wool/silk tucked inside coat	1 briefcase - according to scale and body shape
1 umbrella - black	1 overcoat
	1 raincoat
	1 pair gloves - leather
	1 scarf - wool/silk tucked inside coat
	1 umbrella - black

It's always a good idea to purchase 2 pairs of suit trousers for every jacket. Trousers, especially around the backside, tend to look worn and become shiny more quickly than the jacket.

Also remember to buy your jackets and suits in weights appropriate for the cooler and warmer seasons of the year.

SHOES

Lace up brogues or capped shoes are your best bet with a business suit. You can wear a slip on, including a buckle shoe, as long as the occasion is not too formal. Match your socks, which should be good quality so your feet can breathe, with your shoes or your suit.

MANAGE YOUR WARDROBE

Make your wardrobe work for you. You'll feel so much better when you've done this.

1. Clear the clutter

If you haven't worn it in 2 years, throw it out. Don't think it will be OK when you've lost those extra pounds, got that new job or it comes back into fashion. It's clutter and it needs to go. Anything that is tatty, out of date, too big or too small should be given to your nearest charity shop as soon as possible.

2. Don't waste money

Remember Pareto's rule. When buying new items, make sure they will go with at least 3 other things you already own. Parisian women purchase outfits while both men and women in the UK tend to buy individual garments. They look chic, we may not!

Remember also CPW. The Cost Per Wear of your garment is essential to getting value for your well-earned pound. A designer coat worn every day may cost less per wear than a cheaper one worn twice a year.

3. Store clothes by type

Hang your jackets together and trousers together and so on. This will provide a new and creative way of wearing what you already have. Alternatively, divide your wardrobe into colours so you can easily see what items compliment each other.

4. Buy for your personality

If you like variety, spend less on each item so you can throw it away without guilt. If you like quality, spend more time looking for the right garment and making sure it will last you at least 2 or 3 seasons. If you have a small budget, make sure you spend the money on the accessories. Cheaper clothes with quality accessories will have more positive impact than cheap accessories with good quality tailoring. The golden rule is to make sure whatever you buy fits you and suits you. If you can, take a list of what you require with you when shopping and STICK TO IT! Stay focused so you don't end up with lots more mistakes clogging up your wardrobe space.

5. Hire

It can make sense to hire rather than buy. A dinner jacket can be an expensive purchase if only worn once. Items like these are liable to date when sitting around in the wardrobe, so hiring can ensure you remain current.

6. Enjoy your clothes

Buy wisely and it's one less thing to think about. When you know you look good, you feel good. They are inextricably linked. That means you can concentrate on more important issues, like getting that new business deal.

LOOKING AFTER YOUR WARDROBE

"Fine feathers make fine birds"
Proverbs

Now you've invested all this time, money and effort creating your look, it would be a criminal act if you didn't care for your wardrobe correctly.

Here are some tips that will help your clothes serve you well:

- Don't spend too much money on dry cleaning. It takes the life out of your suit. Instead, hang it outside your wardrobe so it can breathe. Don't wear it on consecutive days, but rotate with another.

- The same applies to your shoes. Rotate pairs daily. Polish and feed them, and have them heeled when required. Use shoe trees to help keep their shape.

- Wash and iron shirts after every wear. If the collar looks grubby or frayed, or if the armpits are yellowing, throw it away.

- Don't attempt stain removal on a silk tie. Take it to a specialist dry cleaner.

- Love your clothes. They will repay the favour many times over.

NOW IT'S UP TO YOU

I hope that you have enjoyed reading this book and it has helped you to discover your own style preferences. Now that you know what suits you, it will be easier to shop, manage your wardrobe, save money and most importantly, make the right impact, wherever you go.

Enjoy being you, and relish the chance to shine.

Good luck!

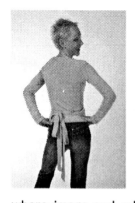

Accentuate – the accent on U, your image and your impact.

Sue Donnelly is an Image Coach with a wide experience of working with people, both in a corporate environment and on a personal basis. She has held a variety of management positions for Thomas Cook, Citibank and Insights Learning & Development where image and relationship building were crucial factors in attracting and retaining business partnerships. Sue's work with individuals enables them to find a style of dress that reflects their inner values and unique personality, elevating self-esteem and confidence. Corporate work includes personal branding seminars and workshops enabling consistency to be reinforced throughout an organisation. She has been featured in national magazines and newspapers, writes a style column for Health Plus magazine, and has been invited to appear on prime time television. She is also the style expert for www.expertsonline.tv and a volunteer for the breast cancer charity, Look Good Feel Better. A qualified life coach, fitness instructor and workshop facilitator with the skills and the passion to help men and women look and feel good about themselves in an authentic way, whatever their age or shape. Her first book, *The 80/20 Makeover*, is also available from www.bookshaker.com

To contact Sue...
Phone: 0845 123 5107
Website: www.thebigu.com

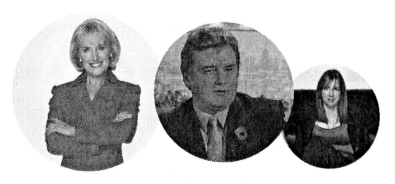

FREE One Year's Subscription To Expertsonline.tv (£70 Value)

As a reader of this book, you are entitled to a free one year subscription to Online TV Channel, Expertsonline.tv worth £70. No catch.

Just go to...
www.passion4business.com/expertsonline
for full details of what the service has to offer and get instant full access with our compliments.

Experience video interviews with the rich, famous and experts in all walks of life, including people like Anita Roddick, Eamonn Holmes, Simon Woodroffe, Rosemary Conley plus many more.

We look forward to welcoming you to our Channel.

expertsonline.tv
The vision to succeed

Style In Motion...

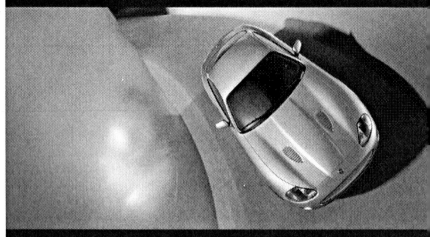

Now you're the epitome of style make sure your car makes a statement too...

At Dove House Jaguar, we offer exceptional quality vehicles with all the main dealer facilities at considerably less than main dealer prices.

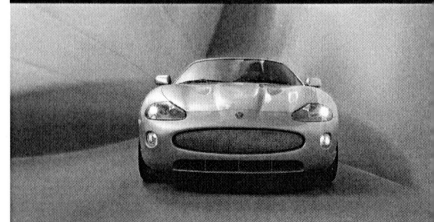

Dove House Jaguar

01733 253 030 | www.dovehousejaguar.com

Dove House   St Pegas Road   Peterborough PE6 7NF

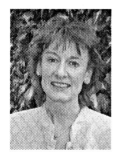
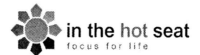

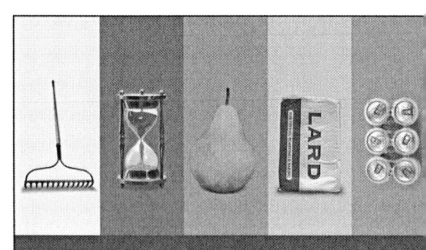
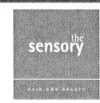

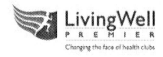

Look The Part

Want to know more about hiding your belly or making the most of your natural assets?

Book a one–to–one with Sue Donnelly and positively transform your image for a more successful, authentic and attractive you.

Colour Analysis

Men's Style

Wardrobe Management

Personal Shopping

Personal Branding

Call now and ask Sue about her range of style and image services just for men…

0845 123 5107

www.thebigu.com

Printed in the United Kingdom
by Lightning Source UK Ltd.
109560UKS00001B/102